THE
BIBLE
CURE ®
FOR

AUTOIMMUNE
DISEASES

DON COLBERT, M.D.

SILOAM

Most Charisma House Book Group products are available at special quantity discounts for bulk purchase for sales promotions, premiums, fund-raising and educational needs. For details, write Charisma House Book Group, 600 Rinehart Road, Lake Mary, Florida 32746, or telephone (407) 333-0600.

The Bible Cure for Autoimmune Diseases
by Don Colbert, M.D.
Published by Siloam
A Charisma Media Company
600 Rinehart Road
Lake Mary, Florida 32746
www.charismahouse.com

Unless otherwise noted, all Scripture quotations are from the Holy Bible, New Living Translation, copyright © 1996, Tyndale House Publishers, Inc., Wheaton, Illinois 60189.

Scripture quotations marked CEV are from the Contemporary English Version, copyright © 1995 by the American Bible Society. Used by permission.

Scripture quotations marked KJV are from the King James Version of the Bible.

Library of Congress Catalog Card Number: 2003113323
International Standard Book Number: 978-0-88419-939-7
E-Book ISBN: 978-1-59979-729-8

This book is not intended to provide medical advice or to take the place of medical advice and treatment from your personal physician. Readers are advised to consult their own doctors or other qualified health professionals regarding the treatment of their medical problems. Neither the publisher nor the author takes any responsibility for any possible consequences from any treatment, action or application of medicine, supplement, herb or preparation to any person reading or following the information in this book. If readers are taking prescription medications, they should consult with their physicians and not take themselves off of medicines to start supplementation without the proper supervision of a physician.

22 23 24 25 26 — 19 18 17 16 15
Printed in the United States of America

A Revelation of Unlimited Love

If you could become fully aware of God's super-natural love for you for even one moment, your life would be changed eternally. That's because God's love for you is far beyond limited human love. He wanted an object of His wonderful love, someone upon whom He could lavish heaven's unlimited, unparalleled love. So, He tenderly created you. (See Deuteronomy 10:15.)

The Bible says that God's love is unfailing, meaning there is nothing you can do to change His tender affection and unwavering compassion toward you. Rest assured that He loves you and cares more for your health than you do.

That's why it is no accident that you've picked up this Bible Cure. I'm convinced that it's part of God's plan for healing and recovery for your life. If you are experiencing the symptoms of an auto-immune disease, or if you have been diagnosed with one, know that it is not a life sentence. With God's help and some natural, God-given wisdom, your complete recovery can occur.

Take comfort that you are not alone in your battle against an autoimmune disease. About 40 million Americans are also contending with some type of autoimmune disease,[1] and there are more than eighty different autoimmune diseases.

You can see we're in the midst of an epidemic of autoimmune diseases, but why? I believe the reasons usually involve a combination of factors. First is poor diet. Second is our poor gastrointestinal health. The third factor involves food sensitivities and allergies with which so many Americans suffer. Fourth, and possibly the most significant factor, is the excessive amounts of stress that most Americans are under. Why are women experiencing far more autoimmune diseases than men? In part, it's because of the vital link between these diseases and hormonal imbalances—which is the fifth factor. The sixth reason for this out-of-control epidemic of autoimmune disease is toxic overload. We are laboring under alarming levels of toxicity in this nation. In addition, many individuals' immune systems must also labor against microorganisms, of which they may be completely unaware—the seventh factor. The final factor is genetics, which you have no control over.

It's easy to see why this is such a mammoth problem in America, and it's growing larger. Nevertheless, autoimmune disease does not have to rob you of the vital health God intended for you to enjoy.

Addressing the Spiritual Roots of Disease

As a Christian medical doctor, I have studied and prayed about the causes of disease, and increasingly I have discovered that many diseases have very strong spiritual roots. If you are familiar with my books, then you are aware that I believe it is God's desire to restore us to complete health of the entire person: body, mind and spirit.

Although traditional medicine often sees these facets of our being as very separate, in truth they are not. A vital link exists between the spirit, soul and body. And although much of the disease and physical pain we suffer comes from the body, often these distresses begin in the spirit and the soul, which encompass the mind and emotions. The Bible says, "The spirit of a man will sustain his infirmity; but a wounded spirit who can bear?" (Prov. 18:14, KJV). I've seen that deep wounds in a person's spirit need to be healed too in order for genuine recovery to take place in the body. Therefore, truly walking in the divine health that God intends for us requires that we look a little deeper, beyond the physical process of disease to the spiritual, emotional and mental roots.

Autoimmune disease can have profound spiritual roots. The Bible encourages us to love others as we love ourselves (Gal. 5:14). Yet, I have seen that self-hatred and internalized regret from an individual's past can link rejection of oneself to autoimmune disease. Although this may be an entirely new concept to you, it may provide a stunning spiritual key to your complete recovery. We'll explore this spiritual link and others, along with a wealth of natural and medical wisdom to bring your body back to vital health.

God desires that we walk in total and complete health. This Bible Cure is filled with hope and encouragement for understanding how to keep your body fit and in a healthy balance. In this book, you will

uncover God's divine plan of health for body, soul and spirit,

*through modern medicine, good nutrition
and the medicinal power
of Scripture and prayer.*

Throughout this book, key Scripture passages will help you focus on the power of God. These divine promises will empower your prayers and redirect your thoughts to line up with God's plan of divine health for you—a plan that includes victory over your autoimmune condition.

This Bible Cure will give you a strategic plan for managing your environment and controlling the triggers of autoimmune diseases in the following chapters:

If you are suffering with an autoimmune disease, take fresh confidence in the knowledge that God is real, that He is alive and that He loves you more than you could ever imagine. You *can*

enjoy complete restoration of your health—
body, soul and spirit.

It is my prayer that these powerful godly
insights will bring health, wholeness and spiritual
refreshing to you. May they deepen your fellowship
with God and strengthen your ability to
worship and serve Him, fulfilling your divine
purpose on the earth.

—DON COLBERT, M.D.

A BIBLE CURE PRAYER FOR YOU

*Father, thank You for Your great love for
me. As I read through the pages of this
book, give me a fresh, living revelation of
Your wonderful love for me. Teach me to
know and trust You in a brand-new way.
Quicken truth and wisdom to my mind,
and give me the strength and determination
to walk out the healing steps I discover
in this book. In Jesus' name, amen.*

Chapter 1

God Is for You

If you are battling an autoimmune disease, the most important thing you can know is that God is on your side, constantly working on your behalf in order to see you well. He desires to see you recover even more than you do. One glimpse of His wonderful love for you would cause you to exclaim as the psalmist: "This I know, that God is for me" (Ps. 56:9, NAS). God is for you.

The word *auto* is from the Greek word meaning "self." When your immune system is operating normally, it identifies, attacks and eliminates foreign or invader cells. But when you have an autoimmune disease, the immune system becomes confused, turning the body's attack against itself. Now the immune system targets certain cells, tissues and organs in your own body.

A normal, healthy immune system can correctly distinguish between self-cells and invader cells or microorganisms. That's because each of our self-cells has an identification code similar to a social security number, called the "human leukocyte antigen," or HLA. The HLA on these self-cells signals the immune system that these cells belong to the body. However, for unknown reasons in autoimmune disease, the immune system mistakenly misreads the HLA code and launches an attack against certain cells, tissues and organs in your own body.

There are many different forms of autoimmune disease, including rheumatoid arthritis, lupus, multiple sclerosis (MS), Crohn's disease, ulcerative colitis, psoriasis, Type 1 diabetes, Graves' disease, Hashimoto's thyroiditis and so forth. In fact, each autoimmune disease involves a different main organ that has come under attack by the confused immune system. For example:

- Multiple sclerosis, autoimmune neuropathies and myasthenia gravis involve an attack on the nervous system itself.
- Psoriasis, vitiligo, dermatitis herpetiformis and pemphigus vulgaris all involve an attack of the skin.
- Lupus, scleroderma, rheumatoid arthritis, polymyositis and Sjogren's syndrome

all affect multiple organs, including the musculoskeletal system.

- Crohn's disease, ulcerative colitis and primary biliary cirrhosis involve an attack on the gastrointestinal tract.
- In pernicious anemia, autoimmune hemolytic anemia and autoimmune thrombocytopenia, the confused autoimmune reaction is directed against the blood.
- Temporal arteritis, Behcet's disease and anti-phospholipid syndrome result when the faulty immune reaction is directed against the blood vessels.
- Graves' disease, Hashimoto's thyroiditis and Type 1 diabetes involve a confused autoimmune reaction directed against the endocrine glands.

As you can see, autoimmune reactions can be directed against the nervous system, gastrointestinal system, blood, musculoskeletal system, endocrine system, skin and even blood vessels.

An Amazing Army

Your immune system commands a 100-million-plus-cell army strategically arrayed in an amazing defense system against disease and other outside invaders. When bacteria or a virus enters your body, the immune system enables your body to fight off the infection.

Healthy immune systems produce antibodies, which are proteins that help to destroy invading organisms such as bacteria and viruses. But when your immune system becomes confused, as with the autoimmune disease lupus, it starts making "autoantibodies." These are self-destructive antibodies sent to attack the body itself.

A Closer Look

Lupus is just one of the many autoimmune diseases that function similarly. Let's turn now and investigate some of the most common autoimmune diseases.

Lupus

Lupus is Latin for "wolf," and like a vicious, wild predator, this disease can tear and destroy your body's health. Three main types of lupus exist.

The first is *systemic lupus* (or *systemic lupus erythematosus*—SLE), which has the potential of impacting almost any organ of the body. Fortunately, most cases of systemic lupus do not affect internal organs. This somewhat

4

less destructive variety is called "non-organ-threatening systemic lupus."

When systemic lupus does affect organs, such as the heart, lungs, kidneys or brain, it is called "organ-threatening systemic lupus." About 35 percent of lupus sufferers fall into this category.

The most common age for the onset of lupus is between the ages of fifteen and forty-five. Eighty to 90 percent of those with lupus will have a normal life span.

Another type of lupus is *drug-induced lupus*. Individuals with this type of lupus develop symptoms after taking certain prescription medications. The main three medications known to cause lupus include:

- *Isoniazid*, used to treat tuberculosis
- *Hydralazine*, used to treat hypertension
- *Procainamide*, used to treat arrhythmias of the heart

More than seventy different medications have been known to trigger drug-induced lupus. Among these are sulfa drugs, penicillin and tricyclic antidepressants. The good news is that this form of lupus is very mild and disappears when the medication is discontinued.

A third type of lupus is *cutaneous lupus* (or *discoid lupus*), which means it affects only the skin. About 10 percent of diagnosed lupus sufferers have discoid lupus.

If you are African American, Latin American, Asian or Native American, you are far more likely to be diagnosed with lupus. The most common symptoms of lupus are joint pain and swelling, fatigue or malaise, and skin rash.

A BIBLE CURE HEALTH TIP

Check Your Symptoms

According to the American College of Rheumatology, the following symptoms may indicate you have lupus. Check the boxes below for any symptoms you might have.

❑ I have a butterfly-type rash over the cheeks.

❑ I have a discoid rash, or raised red patches with scaling and scarring, which usually appear on sun-exposed areas.

❑ I am experiencing photosensitivity as a reaction to sunlight or other types of light such as fluorescent lights.

- ❏ I have oral ulcers such as aphthous ulcers, which are painless lesions on the mouth and resemble cold sores.

- ❏ I have arthritis or swelling and tenderness in two peripheral joints in the arms, legs, feet or hands.

- ❏ I have pericarditis or pleuritis, which is inflammation of the lining of the heart or the lung.

- ❏ I have mild to severe kidney problems.

- ❏ I've been experiencing neurological problems including memory problems, seizures, depression and psychosis.

- ❏ I've had blood abnormalities, including a low white blood cell count, low platelet counts or hemolytic anemia.

- ❏ I've received a positive antinuclear antibodies (ANA) test.

- ❏ I have immunological problems; the presence of anti-DNA, anti-Sm and antinuclear antibodies; a positive test for lupus anticoagulant; or a false positive serologic test for syphilis.

You will need to meet at least four of these eleven criteria before a diagnosis of lupus can be made. However, if you have an ANA test that is strongly positive with a speckled pattern, then it is very likely that you have lupus and should consult with your physician. In addition, most individuals with lupus usually have a positive anti-DNA or anti-Sm antibodies.

Another extremely common and equally distressing autoimmune disease is rheumatoid arthritis. Let's take a look.

Rheumatoid Arthritis

Although many people associate rheumatoid arthritis with pain and swelling in the joints, it's actually a systemic disease that can affect other areas of the body as well. Fatigue, fever and weight loss are very common symptoms during the early stages of the disease. Enlargement of the spleen and lymph nodes may also occur, as well as anemia, pericarditis and lung disease.[1]

Those with rheumatoid arthritis are also at higher risk for developing certain cancers, especially lymphoma.

A Helpful Self-Test

Have you been wondering if you might have rheumatoid arthritis? Carefully consider the symptoms below, and check each one that applies to your own situation.

- ❏ I have morning stiffness that lasts for at least one hour.
- ❏ I have swelling in more than one joint.
- ❏ I am experiencing pain on motion of at least one joint.
- ❏ Symmetrical joints in my body (both knees, both hands, etc.) are swollen. This excludes the joint closest to the fingertips.
- ❏ X-ray findings indicate I have rheumatoid arthritis.
- ❏ I have lumps or nodules under the skin on the forearm.
- ❏ I have received a positive rheumatoid factor test.

According to the Arthritis Foundation, you must have six of the seven criteria to receive a diagnosis of rheumatoid arthritis. In addition, you must have experienced symptoms for the first four criteria longer than six weeks.

Hopefully, the self-test will inform you about the possibility of having rheumatoid arthritis; however, you should also consult with your physician.

Let's turn now to examine one more autoimmune disorder, multiple sclerosis.

Multiple Sclerosis

The actual cause of MS is still unknown. Even though there has been much speculation about possible viruses or toxins as the cause for this disease, no evidence has been found to prove such theories. Yet, multiple sclerosis continues to be a destroyer, impacting the lives of one in seven hundred people in the U.S.

Diagnosing this disease involves locating at least two areas of destruction or scarring in the central nervous system, which includes the brain and the spinal cord. MRI scans have proven helpful in this respect. Yet, multiple sclerosis presents a puzzle that continues to elude the best medical minds.

For instance, it is far more commonly found in northern parts of the Northern Hemisphere and the southern parts of the Southern Hemisphere. These are cooler climates above latitudes at 40 degrees north—from Columbus, Ohio, and Boulder, Colorado—and below 40 degrees south—southern Australia, southern Chile and so forth. MS is far less common in topical climates.

Symptoms of MS include problems maintaining balance, fatigue, muscle spasms and tremors, weakness, bladder and bowel control problems, memory problems and visual problems. Symptoms worsen when exposed to warmer temperatures.

Crohn's Disease and Ulcerative Colitis

Crohn's disease and ulcerative colitis are inflammatory diseases of the gastrointestinal tract. *Inflammation* literally means being "set on fire." And many sufferers of these diseases will tell you that this is exactly how they feel during a flareup.

Crohn's disease can occur anywhere in the body, from the mouth to the anus. It usually occurs at the end of the ileum, which is in the small intestines and the beginning of the colon. Crohn's disease is much more common in women than in men.

> *I show this unfailing love to many thousands by forgiving every kind of sin and rebellion.*
> —EXODUS 34:7

On the other hand, colitis occurs only in the colon and always involves the rectum. Men and women get ulcerative colitis in equal numbers. Interestingly, inflammatory bowel disease is also three times more common in Jews as in non-Jews. It's more often found in developed countries, such as the countries of North America, Western Europe and Scandinavia, and it is more likely to attack individuals in higher socio-economic brackets.

Some type of inflammatory bowel disease affects more than one in five hundred Americans. Some doctors do not classify inflammatory bowel disease as autoimmune since no autoantibodies have been identified. Yet, all agree there is a greater risk of colorectal cancer in patients with Crohn's disease of the colon and individuals who have ulcerative colitis.

A Devastating Impact

Autoimmune diseases are wreaking havoc on more individuals than you might imagine. Psoriasis, an autoimmune disease that attacks the skin, affects two out of every one hundred Americans. Autoimmune thyroid disease affects four out of every one hundred women. Type 1 diabetes occurs in one out of eight hundred people in the U.S. (Read more about these complex diseases in my other Bible Cure books.)

Yet I have discovered that autoimmune diseases can be healed when you remember that God placed within your body a divine disposition toward healing. Healing is as natural as breathing, but the only reason you're staying sick is that something is in the way. I call it a thorn.

Removing the Thorn

When treating autoimmune diseases, I have found that when the thorn—whatever is blocking the body's ability to heal—is removed, the body will usually begin to heal. The "thorn" is usually a combination of factors, including a poor diet, food sensitivities, poor GI tract health, poor digestion, hormonal imbalance, toxic overload, stress and microorganisms to which the immune system may be reacting. Throughout the next several chapters we'll be taking a look at these "thorns" and discovering ways to help you remove them in order to allow God's natural healing streams to flow through your body once more.

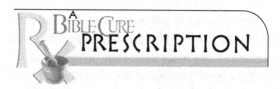

A BIBLE CURE PRESCRIPTION

List any symptoms of an autoimmune disease that you may have.

_____

_____

Have you been diagnosed with an autoimmune disease? If so, which one?

_____

Pray the following prayer, submitting yourself to God.

> *Dear Lord, I submit my body to You, the health of every cell, organ and tissue. I acknowledge You alone as my wonderful, divine Creator. Only You have the divine wisdom to bring my body back to health and wholeness. I place myself in Your hands, and I choose now to trust in Your unfailing love. I receive Your healing power. In Jesus' name, amen.*

Chapter 2

Love Written Over
You—Nutrition

If your eyes were open and you could see God right now, what would you see? Interestingly, Moses wondered about the same question. He asked God to reveal Himself, and the Bible says, "[God] passed in front of Moses and said, 'I am the LORD, I am the LORD, the merciful and gracious God. I am slow to anger and rich in unfailing love and faithfulness'" (Exod. 34:6).

Moses saw a God who loved him, and if your eyes were opened right this moment, that's what you would see, too. In fact, He loves you so much that He's written LOVE in large letters over your head! The Bible says, "He has brought me to his banquet hall, and his banner over me is love" (Song of Sol. 2:4, NAS). All heaven looks down and sees you under the shadow of God's great love for you.

God has numbered the hairs on your head, He hears your anxious thoughts in the dark recesses of the night, and He is eager to respond to every whisper from your heart.

Although you may not see it as such, one expression of God's love in your life is the wonderful array of delicious, healthy, living foods with which He has filled the earth. He really has spread out a banquet before you. (See Genesis 1:29.)

Sadly, much of today's epidemic of autoimmune disease comes from our poor diets. Instead of eating the vital, living foods that God provided for the healthy maintenance of our bodies, our modern diets are primarily made up of dead foods. Dead foods are grains and vegetables that have been devitalized through processing and storage. Let's take a look at dead foods and live foods.

Wanted: Dead or Alive?

Hippocrates, the father of medicine said, "Our food should be our medicine and our medicine should be our food." In other words, the foods we eat should be so good for us that they actually heal and restore our bodies. That's why we need to eat living foods that are rich with vitamins, minerals, enzymes and so much more.

Many years ago my wife, Mary, and I were sitting in a hotel restaurant having breakfast when

I began noticing something that underscores a very powerful truth. This restaurant had two buffet bars filled with everything you could imagine. However, one of the buffet tables was replete with living foods. It was filled with a colorful display of many kinds of wonderful fruits, yogurts, whole-grain breads and cereals. The other buffet offered Danishes, doughnuts, breakfast cakes, white rolls and sugary cereals—all dead foods. As I sat back and watched people survey the two tables of food offerings, I began to notice something amazing.

I turned to Mary and said, "Watch the people who go to each of these breakfast bars, and tell me what you notice."

At first my wife's face looked a little puzzled, but in a few minutes I could almost see a light go on as her face beamed with illumination.

She gasped, "Don, the people who are choosing the dead foods have pasty, sagging skin, puffy faces and dark circles under their eyes."

"And those preferring the live foods..." I added.

She gasped even louder, "They are thinner, with better color and healthier-appearing skin. Why, Don, they look ALIVE while the others look nearly DEAD!"

We both sat there in stunned silence. It was

true; those who chose living food had bodies that radiated vital health and life. Those who selected dead foods had puffy, pale, pasty skin, gray shadows on their faces, dark circles under the eyes, and were generally obese. They really did look half dead.

Mary and I left that restaurant more committed than ever to bringing our message of walking in divine health to the masses.

Take Another Look

Perhaps it is time that you took a closer look at your own dietary choices and consider how they are impacting your overall health. Is your diet rich in an abundant variety of garden-fresh fruits and vegetables? Do you prefer complex carbohydrates to overly refined, processed and bleached carbohydrates?

Think about this for a minute: When I was growing up, my mother had to carefully store flour in airtight containers, and she had to use it up very quickly. That was because flour, even the processed varieties, had a relatively short shelf life. If not stored carefully and used quickly, my mother would open up a container and look inside to find that it was full of bugs and unusable.

That seems like a very unpleasant experience. But has it ever happened to you? Probably not. Do you know why? Because the flour we purchase in the grocery store today has been so overly processed that it no longer contains any nourishment for bugs. Food companies are happy because they

> *But I lavish my love on those who love me and obey my commands, even for a thousand generations.*
> —DEUTERONOMY 5:10

have extended the shelf life of flour and grains to an almost unlimited amount of time. Those who bake with flour have been happy as well because they no longer have to wonder if bugs have ruined their flour.

So, if everyone is happy, what could be wrong? Well, stop for a minute to consider that if the processed flour in your pantry no longer nourishes a bug, neither will it nourish you. Many of today's breads, cakes, rolls, tortillas, buns, cookies and pies are made from flour that has virtually no nutritional value at all. It is almost as dead as the bag of plaster in your garage.

When our daily dietary choices are made up of dead foods, not only are our bodies being denied the vital nutrients they need, but they are also forced to deal with the impact of digesting and eliminating dead foods. And we wonder why we are battling an epidemic of disease in this country. Just imagine what it might do to your body to eat that bag of plaster from your garage every day. It's a mental picture that can make you start thinking about whether you are choosing living foods or dead foods!

Remember, you are alive, and your body is a living organism, which is why it requires living foods.

Finding the Right Balance

God created all living things to live in a careful, delicate state of balance. Your body is no different from any other natural thing. And to be properly maintained, your body requires the right balance of living, healthy foods.

Dr. Barry Sears, author of the best-selling book *Enter the Zone*, says, "Food is the most powerful drug we will encounter."[1] In other words, our bodies are able to react to the foods we receive more powerfully than they react to drugs. That's why we should carefully consider everything we take into our mouths.

This especially applies to individuals with

autoimmune diseases. Sears views virtually every disease today, including autoimmune diseases, as nothing more than the body making more bad super hormones called "eicosanoids" and fewer good ones. According to Sears, *eicosanoids* are "super hormones that control all of the body's hormonal systems and virtually every vital physical function."

Eating the right living diet can help your body maintain a healthy balance of these super hormones. Maintaining a proper balance of proteins, carbohydrates and fats will create the right balance of eicosanoids to control the immune system and even autoimmune diseases. Achieving that balance means that all of your calories would be consumed in the following amounts:

- 40 percent of your calories as complex carbohydrates (not highly processed carbohydrates)
- 30 percent of your calories as protein
- 30 percent of your calories as fats

It's critically important to choose goods fats, unrefined carbohydrates and lean, free-range or organic unprocessed proteins. For more information on how to combine foods properly, I recommend *The Bible Cure for Weight Loss and Muscle Gain.*

Choose Good Fats

You may believe that eating any fat is bad for you. That is simply not true. Eating enough of the right kinds of fat is vitally important for good health. The right balance of essential fatty acids keeps the immune system functioning properly and in balance.

The right kinds of fats make all the difference in the world. So, learn to choose good fats and avoid bad ones. Let's look at these.

Bad fats—omega-6 fatty acids

Omega-6 fatty acids are found in the following:

- Most vegetable oils, salad dressings and fried foods
- Sunflower oil
- Safflower oil
- Corn oil
- Soybean oil
- Cottonseed oil
- Processed and packaged foods

Americans tend to over-consume omega-6 fatty acids. Omega-6 fatty acids tend to stimulate the body's production of many inflammatory chemicals. That means eating too much of these kinds of fats can increase inflammation.

GLA (gamma-linolenic acid)

GLA is one form of omega-6 fatty acid that is very different from the others. This omega-6 fatty acid works to decrease inflammation. It actually behaves more like an anti-inflammatory omega-3 fatty acid.

GLA is derived from evening primrose oil, borage oil and black currant seed oil.

Good fats—omega-3 fatty acids

The average American's diet is generally deficient in omega-3 fatty acids. These are the good fats that are vitally important for maintaining a strong and healthy immune system. Omega-3 fatty acids actually help your body turn off inflammatory reactions, which makes them powerfully important in treating autoimmune disease.

Omega-3 fatty acids are found in oily, fatty fish (such as salmon, mackerel, herring and sardines) and flaxseed oil.

It's critically important to maintain the right balance between omega-3 and omega-6 fatty acids in order to decrease inflammation and to control autoimmune diseases. Eating fatty fish or taking fish oil supplements is the best way to get the omega-3 fatty acid you need.

Flaxseed oil provides these fatty acids also, but for your body to convert it properly requires special enzymes that many people with autoimmune diseases tend to lack. Therefore, I don't suggest attempting to get this good fat by consuming only flaxseed oil.

If you prefer, you may fill your body's needs for these fats by taking omega-3 fats in supplement form. However, much of what is provided at health food stores tends to have a fishy smell, meaning it has become rancid. If you prefer to take supplements, I recommend non-rancid fish oil capsules such as Divine Health Omega-3 Fatty Acids. (See appendix.)

Good fats—omega-9 fatty acids

The omega-9 fatty acids are another very good fat. These can be found in olive oil (especially extra-virgin), avocados, macadamia nuts and almonds. These beneficial fats work together with the omega-3 fats and GLA to decrease inflammation.

From Bad to Worse—Hydrogenated Fats

Hydrogenated fats also have a very long shelf life. Yet, these fats tend to take our health from bad to worse, at least when it comes to eating fat.

Today scientists have learned that partially hydrogenated and hydrogenated fats are far more hazardous to the health than saturated fats, butter and fatty cuts of meat.[2] In addition, these fats tend to interfere with the body's anti-inflammatory compounds, which, in turn, can aggravate autoimmune diseases. You can find these fats in the following:

- Vegetable shortening
- Hard margarine (these are the worst hydrogenated fats)
- Nondairy creamers
- Most salad dressings
- Most baked goods
- Most processed foods (these tend to be made with partially hydrogenated fats)

Avoid canola oil also, since it typically is high in trans fatty acids, which are partially hydrogenated.

If you have an autoimmune disease, stay away from fried foods. Reject fried chicken, french fries, fried catfish, onion rings and all other pan-fried or deep-fried foods.

Deep-fried foods are the worst. They contain high amounts of lipid peroxides. These substances actually create free-radical reactions and encourage inflammation. Instead of fried foods, prefer baked, broiled or grilled selections.

Saturated Fats

Americans consume too many saturated fats, which are found in fatty cuts of meat, the skin of chicken and turkey, and fatty processed meats.

We have approximately 60 to 100 trillion cells in our bodies, and every one of them is encased in a cell membrane containing a mixture of unsaturated and saturated fatty acids. These fatty acids provide strength and flexibility. In addition, nutrients are absorbed in the cells through these membranes. Toxins are also released through the cell membranes.

Most individuals with autoimmune diseases eat large amounts of omega-6 fats, fried foods, hydrogenated fats and saturated fats. These bad fats cause the cell membranes to lose much of their flexibility. When this happens, they cannot absorb nutrients properly or adequately perform the functions for which they were designed.

Yet, limited amounts of saturated fats are important for health. Try to get these fats by eating organically raised free-range meats, chicken and turkey instead of other meats that are generally high in saturated fats.

Fats are critically important for a healthy immune system and in helping to control auto-immune disease.

A BIBLE CURE RECIPE

Treat your health to this delicious salad dressing made with beneficial fats.

1 cup extra-virgin olive oil (cold pressed)

¼ cup balsamic vinegar

2 fresh basil leaves, chopped

1 small clove fresh garlic, crushed

Store in a salad dressing carafe. Shake well before using.

Note: Create your own dressing recipes with olive oil and your favorite spices.

Please Pass the Unprocessed, Unrefined, Complex Carbs

Carbohydrates make up the bulk of what most of us eat every day. Yet, many of us make selections that pack our GI tract with dead, devitalized substances that harm, not heal, our bodies—especially when we're battling autoimmune disease.

If we are ever going to reclaim our good health, we must get off of our refined carbohydrate kick. We eat far too many highly processed, overly refined, devitalized carbohydrates. Here are a few examples of refined carbohydrates you should limit or avoid altogether:

- White bread
- Pasta
- Sugars such as sucrose and high-fructose corn syrup
- Cornstarch
- French fries
- Most breakfast cereals
- Cookies
- Cakes
- Bagels
- Pretzels

Eating large amounts of refined grains and sugars creates more inflammation and causes more symptoms in patients with autoimmune diseases. So, choose unrefined carbohydrates found in whole grains, fruits and vegetables.

Only 9 to 32 percent of Americans consume five daily servings of vegetables and fruit as recommended by the federal government.[3] And many who do, choose potatoes and corn as vegetables, which can actually create more inflammation.

Refined carbohydrates, such as white sugar and white flour as well as corn and potatoes, cause a rapid rise in blood sugar. This causes more insulin to be released from the pancreas. Excess insulin creates more oxidative stress, which, in turn, creates more inflammation and usually aggravates autoimmune diseases.

> *May the LORD be loyal to you in return and reward you with his unfailing love!*
> —2 SAMUEL 2:6

Unrefined carbohydrates generally have a lower glycemic index, meaning they don't cause the blood sugar to rise rapidly. Forty percent of your total caloric intake should be from unrefined carbohydrates, such as whole grains, fruits (not fruit juice) and vegetables.

Breakfast Without Orange Juice?

If you are in the habit of drinking orange juice every day for good health, try eating an orange instead. Orange juice is much higher in sugar content than most people realize. Therefore, if you are battling an autoimmune disease, avoid all fruit juices completely, and substitute your favorite selections with whole fruit instead.

Powerful Protein

Getting enough protein is extremely important for a healthy immune system as well as a balanced hormonal system. If you are like many Americans, you are eating too many carbohydrates and not enough protein. Protein should comprise 30 percent of your daily caloric regimen. In a nation where vegetarianism is becoming increasingly popular, it's vitally important to remember to fill your daily needs for protein.

Protein is a vital basic building material of the body. Amino acids of protein are needed by the body to synthesize DNA, hormones, neurotransmitters and other biochemicals.

In choosing a form of protein, fish is one of

the best sources, but prefer fatty fish. Free-range, organically fed chicken and turkey are far better than other fatty selections of meat. Try to eat no more than three to four ounces of a protein at a meal. Don't eat red meat more than once a week, and make sure it is extra lean and free range or organic.

In addition to eating the right amounts of the right foods to combat autoimmune diseases, it is also vitally important to deal with any food sensitivities you may have.

Food Sensitivities

I have found that the majority of my patients with autoimmune diseases have many sensitivities to various foods. Food allergies can be life threatening. However, food sensitivities or food intolerances are simply adverse reactions to food. These reactions often involve the immune system.

Here is a lineup of the usual suspects linked to common food sensitivities:

- Eggs
- Dairy
- Wheat
- Corn

- Baker's yeast and brewer's yeast
- Tomatoes, potatoes and peppers

Individuals with rheumatoid arthritis often find that eating tomatoes greatly aggravates their symptoms. The same happens in individuals with lupus. Eating certain foods can cause a flareup. That's why it is critically important to identify any food sensitivities you may have and either eliminate these foods or undergo a process to desensitize your body to them.

One of the best tests that I have found to diagnose food sensitivities is the ALCAT test. Your doctor can order this test by calling 1-954-923-2990.

> *Give thanks to the LORD, for he is good! His faithful love endures forever.*
> —1 CHRONICLES 16:34

I also strongly recommend NAET for practically all patients with autoimmune disease. NAET is especially helpful for individuals with food sensitivities since it uses applied kinesiology and acupressure in order to diagnose the food sensitivity, as well as avoidance of the allergen for a period of twenty-five hours in order to treat each food sensitivity. To find a practitioner in your area, I recommend that you visit the Web site at www.naet.com.

Many people with autoimmune disease also have an overgrowth of yeast or candida in the intestinal tract. A simple blood test can determine if you do. I also suggest filling out a yeast questionnaire. If you test positive for candida, it is critically important to follow the candida diet as outlined in *The Bible Cure for Candida and Yeast Infections* and to follow the supplement guidelines outlined in the book.

In addition, one of the best things you can do for your health is to drink enough water. Let's look.

A BIBLE CURE HEALTH TIP

How Much Water?

Here's a good way to find out how much water you really need to drink every day.

Write down your weight _____
Divide that number by 2 _____
Remainder = _____

The remainder is the number of ounces of water you need to drink daily.

Wonderful Water

If you are battling an autoimmune disease or an inflammatory response, it's extremely important to drink enough water every day. The vast majority of those with autoimmune disease are chronically mildly dehydrated. When you get dehydrated, usually your histamine levels become elevated, aggravating autoimmune diseases.

Therefore, never wait until you're thirsty to drink water. I recommend alkaline water from the Alkalizer Water Filter for patients with autoimmune disease. (See appendix.)

Renew Your Commitment

The Bible encourages us all to be doers and not hearers only. So, make up your mind to drink more water, eat living foods, balance your diet, choose good fats and choose a pathway to renewed, radiant health. Most of all, never forget that God is on your side. If you could look up with spiritual eyes, you would see His handwriting in large letters over your head declaring, "I love you!"

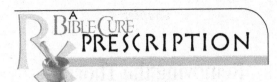

A BIBLE CURE PRESCRIPTION

On a sheet of paper, do the following:

- List ten living foods you eat every day.

- List ten dead foods you plan to stop eating.

- List which healthy fats you will begin using.

Thank God for His great love for you.

Lord, thank You for Your great love for me. Open my eyes every day so that I can readily see that wonderful embrace of Your tender care in and through every detail of my life. Help me to care for this living body You have given me by nourishing it in the way You designed as Creator. Most of all, thank You for a new beginning, a fresh start for renewed health and vitality—body, mind and spirit. Amen.

Chapter 3

Removing the Thorn— Supplements

Wisdom for your healing is found in God. The Bible says, "You are God's children. He sent Christ Jesus to save us and to make us wise, acceptable, and holy" (1 Cor. 1:30, CEV).

In fact, Christ *is* the wisdom of God. And all healing power lies within His wonderful love. No matter what your sickness, you can find complete restoration and wonderful healing in Him—body, mind and spirit.

God's amazing, healing love is expressed for you through the abundance of wisdom He supplies in order to make you well. Too often medical professionals see physical healing in terms of managing symptoms but leaving the root causes unattended. But God knows exactly what your body needs to be completely, totally restored to the vibrant state of health He desires for you to live in.

His wisdom is amazing. And as the divine Creator of your body, He built into it much of His own healing power. That means your body works with divine wisdom in order to heal itself.

Yet, problems come when your body lacks essential materials to complete the healing process. Much like trying to construct a building without nails, your body cannot perform its healing task. Amazingly, however, it will continue to work very aggressively with what it has, trying to accomplish the healing process. It never gives up, and neither does God. He is working right now to bring to light your body's needs, aggressively working to provide you the necessary wisdom to be completely restored.

When your body is laboring to heal itself but lacks certain essential materials to complete the task, the healing stream becomes blocked, much as a dam blocks a river. But when you receive the wisdom you need and give your body what it lacks, the healing streams once again are able to flow freely. Using such healing wisdom is called "removing the thorn." You have taken out the obstruction that was preventing your healing, so now your body is empowered to accomplish the feat it was divinely programmed to do—get well.

Lining Up the Usual Suspects

Supplements are a vital tool for removing the thorn, or providing your body with key materials for healing that it may lack, so that healing can flow freely. Let's examine supplementation of vital materials that may provide some keys to your healing from autoimmune disease.

A comprehensive multivitamin

A comprehensive multivitamin is vitally important to provide the basic vitamins and minerals you need for optimum health. Unfortunately, today's fast-food diet leaves our bodies starving for many essential vitamins and nutrients. And even the fresh fruits and vegetables we eat are often grown in nutrient-depleted soil.

Vitamins and minerals are essential components of your body that it cannot make for itself. It depends upon nutrition for them, but often you cannot get adequate amounts from the food you eat. Therefore, I recommend a comprehensive multivitamin such as Divine Health Elite Multivitamin. It provides essential vitamins and minerals as well as most of the antioxidants your body requires on a daily basis. (See appendix.)

Some individuals with autoimmune disease

may be sensitive to multivitamins and will be unable to take them until they have been desensitized. If you get sick or nauseated when you take a multivitamin, consult a practitioner who can perform NAET. (See S 32.)

Evening primrose oil

In the last chapter, you saw how vitally important getting the right kind of fats is for restoring your body back to health from autoimmune disease. GLA (or gamma-linolenic acid) is a form of omega-6 fatty acid that works to reduce inflammation, much like an omega-3 fatty acid. Evening primrose oil contains GLA.

Take one capsule, three times a day, of Divine Health Evening Primrose Oil. (See appendix.)

Antioxidant formula

It is critically important for individuals with autoimmune disease to supplement their diet with antioxidants on a daily basis. Some of the most important antioxidants are vitamin C, vitamin E, selenium, lipoic acid and coenzyme Q_{10}.

Why are antioxidants so important? The answer is found in understanding the oxidation process. When you cut an apple into slices, what happens? In very short order, the slices turn brown—sometimes in minutes, but always in less than an hour. A good chef will tell you to slow down this process by squeezing lemon juice on the apples.

A similar thing happens to iron. Leave a piece of iron outside for a few months, and it will turn very rusty if it's not specially treated.

What happens to the apples and the iron involves a process called oxidation. The browning of the apples and the rusting of the metal are chemical changes that the naked eye can readily see. However, if you were to purchase a microscope and watch the process at a molecular level, you would see something very different.

> *Because of your unfailing love, I can enter your house; with deepest awe I will worship at your Temple.*
> —PSALM 5:7

You would see tiny particles of matter called electrons spinning freely out of control from their original orbit. These electrons are called "free" radicals because they have been freed from their original position, and they have become oxidized molecules. When these electrons (or radicals) spin freely, other molecules in your body start working to replace them by stealing new electrons from other molecules. Now, chain reactions occur, creating a destructive process that ends up harming or changing the original matter.

This same kind of oxidation process takes place in your body, too. Free radicals create a lot of cellular damage and can eventually damage your DNA. Your DNA contains your genetic thumbprint or code.

Those with autoimmune disease generally have far more inflammation and much more free-radical activity in their bodies. Therefore, taking antioxidant supplements every day is vitally important.

Team antioxidants include vitamin C, vitamin E, glutathione, lipoic acid and coenzyme Q_{10}. Lipoic acid is the only antioxidant that can recycle or restore all the other network antioxidants when they have become depleted. It can even restore itself. Its ability to restore itself as well as other antioxidants makes lipoic acid the captain of the antioxidant team.

Divine Health Elite Antioxidant is a comprehensive formula. I recommend taking one capsule three times a day. (See appendix.)

Sterols and sterolins

Moducare and Natur-Leaf are two different supplements containing sterols and sterolins. These substances are plant fats. Recent research into Moducare has demonstrated that it has potent anti-inflammatory properties.[1]

Sterols and sterolins selectively activate and inhibit the immune system, which provides more effective control to a dysfunctional autoimmune response. Because the average American's diet is generally low in fruits and vegetables, many people lack these sterols and sterolins. Moducare and Natur-Leaf supply them.

To help modulate the immune response and decrease inflammation, I place patients with autoimmune disease on either Moducare or Natur-Leaf. Moducare is available at most health food stores. For information on how to order Natur-Leaf, see appendix.

Warning: Those with MS should not take either Moducare or Natur-Leaf since this may aggravate their condition.

Supplements to Avoid

Some supplements can make autoimmune disease worse. Therefore, it's important to avoid them.

Echinacea

Echinacea is known to boost the immune system, but it can also boost autoantibodies in the immune system, aggravating autoimmune diseases. For those with autoimmune disease, autoantibodies are your enemies. Avoid this herb, especially if you have lupus.

Olive leaf extract and goldenseal

Other herbs that stimulate the immune system, including olive leaf extract and goldenseal, also can aggravate autoimmune diseases, especially lupus. Therefore, avoid these supplements.

Hormonal Imbalance

It's perfectly normal for hormone levels to decline as we age. Yet, most patients with autoimmune disease have extreme hormonal imbalance.

DHEA

DHEA is an adrenal hormone that is considered the mother hormone since it is eventually converted into other hormones such as testosterone, estrogen and progesterone. DHEA is the most prevalent hormone produced by the adrenal glands. Levels of DHEA decline as we age, and most individuals with autoimmune disease have very low levels of DHEA. Using high doses of DHEA in a double-blind study, researchers have found that people with lupus are less likely to suffer exacerbation of their disease than those given placebos.[2] That's why I measure DHEA-S levels. Then I supplement with enough DHEA to get that level up to a normal range.

I recommend pharmaceutical grade DHEA. It's important that you see your physician in order to have your DHEA-S level checked or have salivary hormone testing for DHEA before starting any supplementation. Gradually increase the dose until DHEA levels are adequate.

Testosterone cream

I also usually find testosterone levels to be very low in both men and women with autoimmune disease. Since a whopping 75 percent of all autoimmune diseases involve women, with 90 percent of lupus cases involving women, it is likely that estrogens are involved with these diseases.

Since both men and women need testosterone, I check testosterone levels in all my autoimmune patients. If levels are low or low normal, I supplement them with natural testosterone cream to bring levels back to the normal range.

Progesterone cream

Progesterone is another hormone that's very important in autoimmune disease, especially for women. Progesterone actually is the precursor for cortisol (the stress hormone) and testosterone, as well as estrogens. When an individual's body is under long-term stress, as is the case with most people suffering with autoimmune disease, then the body uses progesterone to make cortisol, which is similar to cortisone.

> *But I trust in your unfailing love. I will rejoice because you have rescued me.*
> —Psalm 13:5

I prescribe natural progesterone cream for most women with autoimmune disease. I generally start with 3 percent progesterone cream and, depending on salivary hormone testing, will increase it to 6 percent and sometimes even 10 percent.

I do not recommend using synthetic progesterones, such as Provera, which can be accompanied by negative side effects, including blood clots, heart attacks and so forth. Natural progesterone cream is free from such side effects.

I recommend *Natural Change Cream* by Nutri-West. (See appendix.) Start by applying

¼ teaspoon twice a day and rotating the sites. I generally recommend using it for three weeks on and one week off. The week off should be during the menstrual period.

For women with MS, it's extremely important to have a progesterone blood or salivary hormone test. Generally, women with MS are very low in progesterone and will need to supplement with progesterone 6 or 10 percent, which can be obtained from a compounding pharmacy. Your physician can prescribe progesterone cream by calling Pharmacy Specialists at 1-407-260-7002.

Natural Thyroid Supplement

Many individuals with autoimmune disease have sluggish thyroid function. It's possible for some cases not to show up on standard thyroid tests. Yet, these individuals have many of the symptoms of hypothyroidism, including low body temperature, intolerance of cold, fatigue, weight gain, loss of one-third of the eyebrows and constipation.

Many individuals with autoimmune disease simply are unable to adequately convert thyroid hormone (T4) to the more active form (T3). If you have symptoms of thyroid disease, please refer to *The Bible Cure for Thyroid Disorders*.

Many individuals with autoimmune disease have low adrenal function. Therefore, I generally place most of my patients on an adrenal glandular formula such as DSF to help support and stabilize the body's stress hormones. The majority of my patients with autoimmune disease benefit dramatically with DSF.

Chew one tablet twice a day, in the morning and at lunch, to supply raw materials to help restore the adrenal function. Occasionally, I have to place a patient on two tablets twice a day. It's extremely important to chew the tablet, even though it doesn't taste good. (See appendix.)

Proteolytic Enzymes

Autoimmune diseases such as rheumatoid arthritis and lupus often respond to systemic proteolytic enzymes. Immune complexes are usually involved in these diseases. These are substances formed when the body attacks what it believes is an outside invader, but in reality, it is attacking itself. These substances, or complexes, attach to tissues in the body, eventually resulting in inflammation and possibly destruction of tissues. Proteolytic enzymes destroy immune complexes.

It's important to take proteolytic enzymes between meals on an empty stomach. I recommend BioZyme from Integrative Therapeutics or Divine Health Proteolytic Enzyme, three tablets twice a day. If you have an autoimmune disease, don't start with three enzymes. Instead, begin with one enzyme twice a day and gradually work up to three. (See appendix.)

If you begin to experience discomfort, burning or nausea when taking these enzymes, stop them. Undergo the following process for healing your GI tract with the supplements before taking these enzymes again.

Repairing the GI Tract

When the lining of the GI tract is healthy, it allows only nutrients from food to pass into the bloodstream. It prevents toxins, bacteria, peptides and partially digested proteins from entering the bloodstream. So you see, a healthy GI tract selectively absorbs nutrients but blocks undesirable substances that could harm us.

Leaky gut syndrome

Occasionally the lining of the GI tract becomes damaged from medications, alcohol, antibiotics, yeast or food sensitivities. This can lead to damage of the intestinal lining and tiny cracks or microscopic holes in the GI tract that allow toxins to pass directly into the circulating blood. When undigested food particles, bacteria and toxins from the bowel leak directly into the bloodstream, it's called *increased intestinal permeability*, or "leaky gut syndrome."

Leaky gut is extremely common in most patients with autoimmune disease. Symptoms of leaky gut are very similar to irritable bowel syndrome and include bloating, gas, abdominal pain, abdominal swelling, irregular bowel function and mucus in the stool. However, symptoms of leaky gut may not be limited to the GI tract. Symptoms may involve the entire body. Autoimmune diseases are usually associated with leaky gut syndrome.

Toxins absorbed from a leaky gut can overwhelm your liver, which is your detoxification organ, and cause many health problems. So you can see that it's vitally important to heal your intestines and repair the leaky gut.

To repair the lining of the GI tract, I recommend a supplement called Total Leaky Gut from Nutri-West. It contains supplements to heal the lining of the GI tract. I recommend chewing one tablet thirty minutes before each meal. (See appendix.)

Probiotic Pearls

About 60 percent of our immune system is located in the GI tract. Repairing the GI tract, as well as replacing the good bacteria, is critically important for maintaining a smoothly functioning immune system.

You may be unaware that about four hundred different species of microorganisms exist in your large intestines. Renowned internist Dr. Leo Galland claims that we have approximately 100 trillion bacteria in our large intestines.[3] It is also believed that we have about three pounds of bacteria in our large intestines.[4] Some of these bacteria are beneficial, but some are not.

Maintaining a healthy balance of good bacteria is extremely important for those with autoimmune disease. Therefore, supplementing with beneficial bacteria is critically important to restore the population of beneficial bacteria to the GI tract. I strongly recommend the supplement Probiotic Pearls by Integrative Therapeutics.

Take one tablet twice a day. The advantage of this product is that it can be taken with meals. (See appendix.)

Digestive enzymes

I also find that the majority of my patients who suffer from autoimmune disease have poor digestion and usually benefit from supplementation of digestive enzymes. Digestive enzymes contain lipase, trypsin and amylase, which help to break down fats, proteins and carbohydrates to fatty acids, amino acids and simple sugars for improved absorption. One of my favorite enzymes is Similase from Integrative Therapeutics. I recommend one tablet three times a day with meals. (See appendix.)

Getting Started…

Many supplements are genuinely helpful for treating autoimmune disease. But you may be wondering, "Where do I start?" I've discovered that the vast majority of individuals suffering from autoimmune disease can begin by taking only a few supplements to start with. Therefore, to simplify matters, I suggest starting off with the following supplementation regimen:

- *Total Leaky Gut:* Start with Total Leaky Gut to heal your GI tract. Chew one tablet thirty minutes before each meal.

- **Probiotic Pearls:** Then begin taking beneficial bacteria, such as Probiotic Pearls. Take one tablet twice a day.

- **Omega-3 fatty acids and evening primrose oil:** Next, start supplementing with omega-3 fatty acids and evening primrose oil. Take one tablet three times a day of each.

- **Moducare or Natur-Leaf:** Moducare or Natur-Leaf is needed to regulate the immune system. I recommend two tablets of Moducare three times a day, one hour before meals. Or, you may choose two tablets of Natur-Leaf twice a day, one hour before meals. However, if you have MS, do not take this supplement.

- **Progesterone cream:** For women, I recommend a natural progesterone cream such as Natural Change Cream from Nutri-West. Apply ¼ teaspoon two times a day.

- **DHEA:** Start with one 5-mg tablet twice a day. Allow it to dissolve in your mouth.

- **DSF:** To help to restore adrenal function

I recommend DSF. Chew one tablet twice
a day at morning and at lunch.

Start your initial supplement program with
these products, then plan to undergo NAET ses-
sions to control food sensitivities, which will
enable you to take more supplements.

Later, antioxidants, multivitamins, proteolytic
enzymes and digestive enzymes may be added. I
also recommend that you supplement with a natural testosterone cream and thyroid supplementation if your lab tests are low.

Tools for Removing the Thorn

I realize that this is a tremendous amount of
information for such a small book. But if you
can begin starting slowly, you will be able to
remove the "thorn" so that your body can heal.

The tools given to you in this book, as well
as the promises in God's Word, should help you
to achieve your goal. Again, I recommend that
you be under the care of a medical doctor. Do
not stop taking your medicines until your doctor
gives you permission.

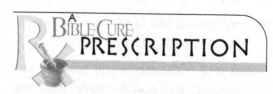

A BIBLE CURE PRESCRIPTION

Has a doctor diagnosed you as having an autoimmune disease? If so, pray the following prayer:

Dear Lord, thank You for creating my body as a complex, powerful, wonderful living being. Moreover, thank You for providing wisdom and understanding as a wise Creator to help me release the healing virtue You have already placed within my body. I truly am fearfully and wonderfully made, just as it says in Your Word. You will show me the "thorns" that are hindering my healing, and You will provide all the insight, understanding, discipline and provision I need to begin walking in Your wonderful divine health. Amen.

Chapter 4

Everything About You Is Important— Exercise and Lifestyle

Everything about you is extremely important to God, even the pain and difficulty you are experiencing because of an autoimmune disease. God cares very deeply about you, even about your pain, discouragement, disappointment and daily struggle. His powerful Word says, "I will seek the lost, bring back the scattered, bind up the broken, and strengthen the sick" (Ezek. 34:16, NAS). So you see, He is more committed to your total recovery than you are!

So why not determine to be as committed to your wellness as God is? Since He also promises in Philippians 2:13 that He will work in you both to will and to do His good pleasure, you have no excuse. He will help you be willing, even when it's a struggle. And if you've tried and tried to exercise while battling an autoimmune disease, you know that getting God's help to stay with it is a must.

The Importance of Exercise

Exercise is critically important for anyone with autoimmune disease, but especially individuals with rheumatoid arthritis, lupus and any autoimmune disease that involves the musculoskeletal system. Exercise can keep joints flexible and ease pain and stiffness. It also helps to strengthen muscles, which help support and protect your joints. Exercise helps to prevent fatigue, and it helps prevent bone loss, which could lead to osteoporosis. Finally, it helps to combat depression and improve your sense of well-being.

Range of motion

Range of motion exercises help to maintain normal joint mobility, prevent stiffness and improve flexibility. If you are battling lupus or rheumatoid arthritis, it's critically important to gently put your joints through their full range of motion at least once a day. These joints include your neck, shoulders, elbows, wrists, fingers, back, hips, knees, ankles and toes.

Stretching

Stretching exercises are also important to improve flexibility and maintain normal joint mobility. Stretches must be done slowly and steadily without bouncing so as not to aggravate inflammation.

Both range of motion exercises and stretching exercises can be performed as a warmup prior to starting aerobics or strength training. For most individuals with chronic rheumatoid arthritis, lupus or other autoimmune disease, range of motion exercises and stretching exercises may be all you should do until your body begins to heal.

Aerobic exercise

As your body heals and your autoimmune symptoms subside, you will find that you can gradually begin incorporating both aerobic exercise and strengthening exercises. Aerobic exercise helps to improve cardiovascular fitness and overall well-being. Aerobic exercise includes walking, cycling, swimming and rowing.

If you are battling an autoimmune disease that has attacked your joints, I recommend you do aerobic exercises that are easy on the joints. A recumbent stationary bike provides a great workout for those with rheumatoid arthritis and lupus. If your inflammation is severe, start at low intensity for a short period of time—two to five minutes. If joint pain or swelling increases, stop your exercise program for that day.

However, prior to starting any aerobic exercise program, I also recommend that you get medical clearance from your doctor. If you experience any chest pain while exercising, stop immediately and consult your physician.

Strength-training exercises

Eventually you will want to begin strength-training exercises. I strongly recommend that you get a physical therapist or a certified personal trainer who is able to demonstrate each exercise and make sure you are performing it properly. Strength training will help to increase muscle mass to help to support and protect your joints.

The Benefits Go On and On

The benefits of a good exercise program are endless and well worth the cost in time, money and effort. Exercise also decreases stress and anxiety by enabling you to burn off stress chemicals that fuel anxiety. It increases endorphins, which help to elevate your mood.

Improved cardiovascular health gained

through regular exercise increases your energy level and promotes restful sleep. In summary, few things do more to promote good health than adequate physical exercise. If you are battling an autoimmune disease, regular exercise is a must!

Our Dirty Planet

The bodies of most of my patients with autoimmune disease are also overburdened with toxic chemicals and heavy metals. Sadly, everyone who lives on Planet Earth has heavy metals as well as solvents stored in their tissues.[1]

Some researchers estimate that we have more than 100,000 chemicals in our environment, with thousands being added each year. We are exposed to pesticides and even DDT, though it was banned decades ago. We are also exposed to secondhand smoke and formaldehyde from carpets and upholstered furniture. Nearly everyone has some lead stored in his or her body.[2]

Heavy metals and solvents create free radicals in the body, generating inflammation and setting the stage for autoimmune disease. These toxic substances also make autoimmune disease much worse. Heavy metals include lead, mercury, arsenic, cadmium, nickel, aluminum and so forth.

One of the most common toxins we are exposed to is mercury. The U.S. Department of Health and Human Services listed mercury as the third most hazardous substance known to man.[3]

One of the main sources of mercury toxicity is dental amalgams, or silver fillings. Amalgams contain 50 percent mercury, and they also contain silver and nickel. Mercury is released as mercury vapor when you chew, especially when you chew gum. If you are battling an autoimmune disease, I recommend you have your amalgam fillings removed by a biological dentist. To find a biological dentist, I recommend you call the International College of Integrative Medicine at 1-419-358-0273.

> *The LORD thy God in the midst of thee is mighty; he will save, he will rejoice over thee with joy; he will rest in his love, he will joy over thee with singing.*
> —ZEPHANIAH 3:17, KJV

You are exposed to mercury by eating fish, especially swordfish, shark and tuna. Water- and oil-based paints usually contain mercury, as well as certain immunizations, some cosmetics and certain pesticides.

In today's world, autoimmune disease isn't all our bodies must battle. Each day they must contend with the contamination of our dirty planet. For more information on this topic, please refer to my books *What You Don't Know May Be Killing You* and *Toxic Relief*.

In addition to chemical toxins, our bodies are also waging warfare against biological toxins too small for us to see.

A Microscopic Menace

We now know that individuals with rheumatoid arthritis, lupus, ankylosing spondylitis, scleroderma dermatomyositis and polymyositis may have Mycoplasma, which is a bacterium without a cell wall.

To find out if your body is battling these microscopic organisms, you will need to have a blood test for Mycoplasma. If it proves positive, consult your primary care physician to begin the antibiotic Minocin, 100 mg every other day.

For those with MS, I also check a blood test for Human Herpes Virus 6 (HHV-6). You may also benefit from Transfer Factor. Transfer Factors are tiny protein molecules that are produced by T-cells, which are immune cells. They allow the immune system to remember conditions for which immunity has already been established.

All mammals produce Transfer Factors. Transfer Factors are able to be produced for specific viruses and bacteria, including HHV-6 and Mycoplasma. For more information, visit the Web site www.immunesupport.com.

I believe that at the root of most autoimmune diseases is toxicity from chemicals and heavy metals, especially mercury, but also to a lesser extent lead, cadmium, arsenic and so forth. I also believe that excessive exposure to chemicals—including pesticides, formaldehyde, toluene and so forth—overburden and confuse our immune system, leading to autoimmune diseases. A very reliable method to test for heavy metal toxicity is urine challenge testing using a chelating agent such as DMSA or DMPS. Physicians may also use the chelator EDTA in addition to one of the chelators above. To find a doctor knowledgeable in chelation, call 1-800-LEADOUT.

For individuals with chemical toxicity, I recommend infrared sauna treatments. Your body will produce up to three times more perspiration with infrared, which helps rid the body of chemical toxins. MS patients may not be able to use a sauna since symptoms generally worsen with heat. For more information on infrared saunas, see the appendix.

Individuals with Crohn's disease should get a blood test for Mycobacterium avium paratuberculosis, or MAP. If you test positive, you will need to be treated with antibiotics.

However, when taking antibiotics, it's extremely important to follow the candida diet, take beneficial bacteria and take Nystatin or herbs to suppress candida overgrowth.

He Cares for You

If you have struggled with exercise regimens in the past, or if you feel intimidated by all of this information about toxins and microorganisms, don't despair. God's power can help you. Ask Him to help you, and He will. The Bible says, "Give all your worries and cares to God, for he cares about what happens to you" (1 Pet. 5:7).

Give Him your discouragement, your hopelessness, your sense of defeat and your lack of control. When you blow it, give it all back to Him again. You will be amazed at how much help you will receive. He is a great and wonderful heavenly Father, and nothing is too difficult for Him! (See Jeremiah 32:27.)

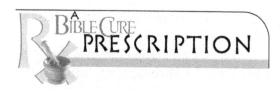

In the box below, outline an exercise program that you are committed to starting right away.

	Range of Motion	Stretches	Aerobic Exercises	Strength Training
Frequency				
Type of exercise(s)				
Time of day				

Dear Jesus, I cast all my care, concern, worry, fear and lack of control upon You right now. Let me exchange my weakness for Your power, my fear for Your courage, my lack for Your control. I give You my disease, and I receive Your healing touch. Amen.

Chapter 5

Loving Yourself and Matters of the Heart

D o you ever wish your eyes could be opened to look directly into heaven? It happened to the apostle John. Here's what he saw: "And he showed me a river of the water of life, clear as crystal, coming from the throne of God and of the Lamb, in the middle of its street. And on either side of the river was the tree of life, bearing twelve kinds of fruit, yielding its fruit every month; and the leaves of the tree were for the healing..." (Rev. 22:1–2, NAS).

The Book of Revelation is a book of symbols that reveal unseen spiritual truths. In it we discover that healing is found in God's wonderful presence. Whenever you experience His presence, you also experience His healing touch. John saw that healing flowed directly from God's glorious throne. If your eyes were open today, you would see that river—an endless healing fountain of love that flows to you from the heart of God.

Throughout this book I have spoken a great deal about God's love for you—for a very good reason. Love is a key element in receiving your healing from autoimmune disease. Many individuals with autoimmune disease do not know how to receive and experience God's deep, unfailing love for them because they have never learned to love themselves. Jan* was one of those people. Here's her story.

Jan's Battle With Lupus

Jan was a thirty-four-year-old woman who came into the office a few years ago with symptoms of severe fatigue and mild joint aches in her fingers and wrists. She lived in Florida, and any time she went to the beach, she would get sunburned, especially over her cheeks and nose. The sunburn would take weeks to go away.

Jan had seen many doctors and received a confusing array of diagnoses. One told her she was suffering with depression and placed her on antidepressant medicine. Another doctor said she had chronic fatigue.

* Not her real name; composite of several different patients

A standard part of treatment at our wellness center involves thoroughly discussing any emotional circumstances that might have influenced a patient's present condition. Jan's story was very difficult to hear.

A couple of years prior to developing her symptoms she had gone through a terrible divorce, lost her job and had a miscarriage. To make matters even worse, she lost the custody of her only daughter. As a result, Jan plummeted into a dark, deep well of depression. She told me that at one point she hoped she would die.

A blood test revealed Jan had a positive ANA, speckled pattern. Another test, an anti-DNA antibody test, confirmed my diagnosis. Jan had lupus.

I'm convinced that the severe stress Jan was under for about two years preceding the onset of her symptoms was the primary reason she developed this autoimmune disease. In effect, Jan had flipped her body's self-destruct switch, and her own immune system started attacking her body.

The Searing Process of Long-Term Stress

As with Jan, a surprising number of autoimmune disease cases are preceded by extremely stressful situations. When stress is left unchecked, it produces a perpetual release of the stress hormones adrenaline and cortisol. These powerful hormones can sear the body in a way that's similar to acid searing metal. Hours after a particularly stressful event has subsided, stress hormone levels can remain high and continue to do their damaging work.

When long-term emotional stress continues and reaches chronic levels, the results of the continual production of these hormones become even more destructive. Now the body begins to damage itself. Like powerful acid pouring into your delicate body systems, the ongoing infusion of chemicals injures tissues and organs. The result can take many different disease forms. This often is how autoimmune disease begins.

> *So let all thine enemies perish, O LORD: but let them that love him be as the sun when he goeth forth in his might.*
> —JUDGES 5:31, KJV

Since autoimmune disease often has destructive emotional and spiritual roots, treating it involves understanding and learning how to yank up these roots.

Learning to Love You

My patients who battle autoimmune disease often are extremely loving individuals when it comes to everyone else. But when it comes to loving themselves, many are completely clueless.

If you are battling autoimmune disease, you may need to learn to love yourself, receive God's love and accept the love and approval of others. This is a critical spiritual root in many autoimmune diseases. Some of us have been wrongly taught that it's incorrect to love ourselves. We are not to live self-centered lives; however, loving ourselves is directly linked to receiving the love of God and others—and it is very biblical.

In Mark 12:31, Christ mentions the second most important commandment: "Love your neighbor as yourself." This commandment assumes the godly kind of self-love, not the kind that's selfish and egotistical. When we are commanded to love our neighbor as we love ourselves, we are actually commanded to love ourselves.

However, many people with autoimmune disease no longer love themselves, but actually hate and despise themselves. When this occurs, the immune system gets conflicting messages. The brain sends messages to the body telling it to hate itself. The brain produces chemical messengers called "neuropeptides" that communicate to the immune cells all over the body. Conversely, these chemical messengers also allow the immune system to communicate back to the brain.

But when the brain is saying, "I hate myself" or "I despise myself," the immune system gets confused and may actually begin to attack itself. It's similar to flipping a self-destruct switch.

That's why it is so critically important to begin to change the message that the brain is giving the immune system by reprogramming your own thoughts. I strongly advise anyone with autoimmune disease to read *The Bible Cure for Stress* and my book *Deadly Emotions*, which addresses this very important issue of loving yourself and decreasing your stress so that your body can heal.

Get a Grip on Destructive Self-Communication

Here's a powerful exercise that will allow you to stop rejecting yourself and begin seeing yourself through God's eyes.

Take note of destructive self-talk and self-messages

One of the most important ways to start

turning off the spiritual switch that is sending self-destructive messages to your immune system is to begin listening to yourself. Discern destructive self-talk and negative self-messages.

They often sound like this:

- "I hate myself."
- "Can't I ever get anything right?"
- "I'm so stupid!"
- "Can't I ever just shut up?"
- "I'm so fat!"
- "I'm so ugly!"

You will know you have entered into a self-destruct pattern if you've ever stood in front of a mirror and spoken abusively or yelled slander at yourself. Most people who do such things would never speak in this manner to anyone else for fear of destroying someone's self-esteem. Yet, they are actively destroying their own.

Stop and apologize to God

When you communicate to yourself in such an abusive fashion, you are sinning against God. He created you, and when He finished the job, He judged it. The Bible says, "And God saw all that He had made, and behold, it was very good" (Gen. 1:31, NAS).

71

The Bible also says that God created you in His own image. "And God created man in His own image, in the image of God He created him; male and female He created them" (Gen. 1:27, NAS).

When you are being so hateful in your thoughts and words toward yourself, you are despising what He has approved. You are judging to be evil what God has already judged to be good. You are grievously sinning against God and yourself. And this is a very, very serious matter.

Whenever you hear yourself speaking or communicating destructive, negative self-talk, stop dead in you tracks and apologize to God.

Look in the mirror and apologize to yourself

This next step may seem a little silly at first, but bear with me. It can produce powerful results. Think for a minute of your own heart as though it were a little child whom you need to protect. I want you to stand in front of a mirror and apologize to yourself for communicating negative, hurtful thoughts and words.

This stressful world in which we live tends to treat us like machines until we start treating ourselves like machines. We forget that we're sensitive, spiritual creatures created in the awesome image of God. We get so caught up in disciplining ourselves and making increasingly strong demands upon ourselves that we lose sight of who we really are.

Stand in front of the mirror and tell yourself you're sorry for all of the times you abused yourself and communicated abusive words, thoughts and emotions to yourself. Apologize for not caring for yourself as you should have done. Repent to your body for not caring for it and cherishing it as a gift from God.

Many of us have been angry with ourselves for years, or we have condemned ourselves for sins dating back twenty years or sins that happened this morning. Look in the mirror and forgive yourself for all of it. Now make a commitment to yourself to be nicer to you.

Broken vows

How many times have you promised yourself you would go on a diet but then broke your promise when a tempting dessert or distressful hunger pang came your way? Someone once said that at times we can't regain control because we have broken so many vows to ourselves that we have lost confidence in ourselves.

Have you ever promised God you would do

something, and then blew it off when it became difficult? Perhaps you made a commitment in church to tithe, but felt tempted to spend the allocated funds on a new dress.

These are broken vows to yourself and to God. Such broken promises can cause us to place ourselves under a self-inflicted prison of condemnation. In order to be free, ask God to forgive you for any vows to Him you've broken, even those you can't remember. Now, stand and look in the mirror and repent to yourself as well.

Overcoming Bitterness

I am also convinced that prolonged bitterness can lead to autoimmune disease. I have witnessed many patients who have gone through a bitter divorce and harbored bitterness and hatred in their hearts toward their ex-spouse. Within a few years many of these individuals, especially women, go on to develop an autoimmune disease.

Matthew 6:14–15 says, "If you forgive those who sin against you, your heavenly Father will forgive you. But if you refuse to forgive others, your Father will not forgive your sins."

But you may say, "I can't forgive him! He hurt me and my children, and he deserves to suffer."

To forgive does not mean that a person is saying, "This didn't matter." Or, "This wasn't a huge wrong committed against me." Rather it is saying, "I choose to no longer hold this feeling of unforgiveness toward the person who hurt me." It isn't easy, but with practice and patience, the Holy Spirit can gently lead you through the process. Bitterness is like drinking poison and wishing the other person would die. Refer to my book *Deadly Emotions* for more information.

Grieving the Holy Spirit

Now, there's one more unexpected individual with whom I want you to make things right. Although you can't see Him, He is as close to you as your next breath. The Holy Spirit was sent to you by God when Christ ascended into heaven. He has been with you ever since you made a commitment to walk with God. Yet, many of us have grieved this gentle Third Person of the Trinity. The Bible warns us about doing so.

It says, "Don't make God's Spirit sad" (Eph. 4:30, CEV). How do we do that? The Holy Spirit is sad when we hold anger, revenge, bitterness or any other unloving emotion toward someone else. (See Ephesians 4:31–32.)

Take a moment right now and ask the Holy Spirit to forgive you for all the times you have grieved Him. It may be that once a long time ago you felt His presence all the time. But over time, that presence has faded. Perhaps you grieved Him and didn't know it. Talk to Him right now and make it right.

The Antidote to a Lie

Just as antiserum is the antidote to a poisonous snakebite, the truth is the antidote to a lie. From now on, determine to apply the truth to negative, destructive self-talk communications.

> *Thou tellest my wanderings: put thou my tears into thy bottle: are they not in thy book?*
> —PSALM 56:8, KJV

When old patterns of negative self-talk rise up in your mind, have a few scriptures memorized or close at hand to use to combat them. If you hear your heart repeat messages of self-hatred and self-rejection, stop and correct those thoughts with the Word of God.

For instance, "Oh, I hate myself! I hate the way I look."

Stop and count to ten. Now, speak aloud: "God said everything He made was good. He loves me and accepts me."

76

The same is true with negative emotions. Whenever you feel rejected or abandoned due to the words or actions of others, stop. Count to ten. Speak the truth of God about yourself aloud. "God loves me dearly. I am accepted in the Beloved."

There are scriptures placed strategically throughout this book that you can use as truth antidotes to hateful or abusive self-messages.

Messages From Others

If someone walked up to you and handed you a bag of cow dung, would you receive it? Of course not. You would walk away. Well, when life hands you hatred, rejection and abuse, don't receive it. Walk away. Guard your heart from receiving them. The Bible says, "Keep thy heart with all diligence; for out of it are the issues of life" (Prov. 4:23, KJV).

Conversely, if you are like many people with autoimmune disease, you may be a pro at receiving negative messages from others. At the same time, you may have perfected your ability to deflect or reject messages of affirmation and love.

When your spouse, a co-worker or a family member says something nice or encouraging, you shrug off the comment or you disagree with it. A woman may say, "I don't really look good in this dress. It makes me look fat."

A man may say, "I didn't really improve on my golf game as much as I should have."

These are ways we push away the praise, affirmation and love that come our way. If you are a master at deflecting the positive and receiving the negative, you need to repent. It's a sin against yourself and against God. Consider for a minute that God is sending you those positive, kind, affirming words through the lips of someone else. You have no right to reject them.

The next time you hear yourself begin to reject positive words of love and affirmation, stop yourself. Count to ten. Repent silently to yourself, and then smile widely and say, "Thank you!"

That's it. Not "I'm really fat" or "I should have done better." A simple thank you is all that is required. Then as you go on your way, why not whisper a little prayer: "Thank You, God, for that nice compliment. I love You, too."

You and You Alone

Only you can pull down the wall of self-rejection. It may take a little time and work, but it will be well worth it in the long run. Harsh self-judgments, negative self-talk and self-condemnation are spiritual thorns that must be removed for total healing to flow—body, mind and spirit. As you begin to reprogram your mind and heart with the truth, you will discover that God's healing love will flow to you and through you.

The Power of a Merry Heart

Years ago, I had been in practice only a few years and had already treated quite a few patients with rheumatoid arthritis, lupus, MS and numerous other autoimmune diseases. I heard of an unusual evangelist who had a ministry of laughter. People would attend his meetings and be overcome with joy and laughter.

Some of my patients with autoimmune diseases attended his meetings and came back filled with joy and overflowing mirth. When they came to my office for a checkup, I learned that they had stopped taking their medications. Their painful, distressing symptoms had completely disappeared. That was when I discovered the power of laughter and joy in overcoming autoimmune diseases.

Proverbs 17:22 says, "A cheerful heart is good medicine." I am convinced that laughter is one of the best medicines—and it's totally free. How

79

often I see that those who suffer from autoimmune diseases have stopped laughing completely. They live a heavy, glum, painful existence. Laughter actually balances the autonomic nervous system, which allows the body to begin to heal.

Therefore, my final Bible cure prescription for you is this: Learn to laugh often and regularly, and learn to laugh at yourself. Enjoy at least ten belly laughs every day to combat autoimmune disease. And most importantly, never forget how much God loves you!

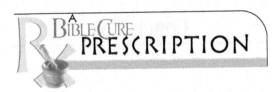

A BIBLE CURE PRESCRIPTION

Pray the following prayer as you ask for God's help.

Lord, deliver me from self-hatred, self-rejection, self-loathing and self-criticism. I repent for every word and thought of self-criticism and self-condemnation that I've internalized and used against myself to wound my own spirit. I repent and renounce the emotions and attitudes connected with those sins. Forgive me and wash me this day. Make me into one who shines brightly with the radiant joy of a healthy, whole and loving spirit. Amen.

Conclusion

The Bibles says that God "satisfies your years with good things, so that your youth is renewed like the eagle" (Ps. 103:5, NAS). With faith in God as well as these practical Bible cure steps, I believe He will empower you to soar above every symptom of autoimmune disease.

With God's help, commit yourself to the nutritional and lifestyle changes outlined here. More importantly, keep your eyes on God as your source of healing, hope, restoration and renewal. Remember that His love for you is as great as God Himself!

—Don Colbert, M.D.

Appendix

Divine Health Products

Call 1-407-331-7007 or visit the Web site at www.drcolbert.com for Divine Health Elite Multivitamins, Divine Health Evening Primrose Oil, Divine Health Divine Health Omega-3 Fatty Acids, Divine Health Elite Antioxidant and Divine Health Proteolytic Enzyme.

Alkalizer Water Filter

E-mail info@alkalizer.com. DBS, Inc. is offering Dr. Colbert's readers a $100 discount on the unit. Mention this code when ordering: DC7007.

Natur-Leaf

Call 1-888-532-7845. Lifeline Inc. is offering a discount to readers of Dr. Colbert's Bible Cures. Provide reference code "Colbert" when placing an order.

Natural Change Cream; DSF; Total Leaky Gut

Call Nutri-West at 1-800-451-5620.

BioZyme; Probiotic Pearls; Similase

Call Integrative Therapeutics at 1-800-931-1709. Use Dr. Colbert's code of PCP-5266.

Infrared saunas

Call QCA Spas and/or TheraSauna at 1-563-359-3881 or visit their Web site at www.qcaspas.com.

A Personal Note From
Don and Mary Colbert

God's Word is full of promises that confirm His love for you and His desire to give you His abundant life. His desire includes more than physical health for you; He wants to make you whole in your mind and spirit as well through a personal relationship with His Son, Jesus Christ.

If you haven't met our best friend, Jesus, we would like to take this opportunity to introduce Him to you. It is very simple. Just bow your head and sincerely pray this prayer from your heart:

> *Lord Jesus, I want to know You as my Savior and Lord. I believe You are the Son of God and that You died for my sins. I ask You to forgive me for my sins and change my heart so that I can be Your child and live with You eternally. Thank You for Your peace. Help me to walk with You so that I can begin to know You as my best friend and my Lord. Amen.*

If you have prayed this prayer, we rejoice with you in your decision and your new relationship with Jesus. Please contact us at pray4me@charisma media.com so that we can send you some materials that will help you become established in your relationship with the Lord. You have just made the most important decision of your life. We look forward to hearing from you.

Notes

Preface

1. "Fulvic Acid Minerals Information," Info Archive Site, http://www.info-archive.com/fulv%20arthritis.htm (accessed December 12, 2003).

CHAPTER 1

1. Eugene Braunwald, et al., ed., *Harrison's Principles of Internal Medicine*, 15th edition (New York: McGraw-Hill, 2001).

Chapter 2

1. Barry Sears, *Enter the Zone* (New York: Harper Collins, 1995.
2. W. C. Willet, et al., "Intake of Trans Fatty Acids and Risk of Coronary Heart Disease Among Women," *Lancet* 341 (March 6, 1993): 581–585.
3. Jack Challem, *The Inflammation Syndrome* (Hoboken, NJ: John Wiley & Sons, Inc., 2003).

Chapter 3

1. I. Louw, et al., "A Pilot Study of the Clinical Effects of a Mixture of Beta-Sisterol and Beta-Sisterol Glucoside in Active Rheumatoid Arthritis," *Am J Clin Nutr* 75 (2002): 351S (Abstract 40).
2. Ibid.
3. Leo Galland, *Power Healing* (New York: Random House, 1997).
4. Ibid.

Chapter 4

1. "Lead, Arsenic, Cadmium—How to Unburden Yourself," Gordon Research Institute, http://www.gordonresearch.com/Lead_Articles/lead_arsenic_cadmium_sinatra.html.
2. Ibid.
3. ATSDR/EPA Priority List, Agency for Toxic Substances and Disease Registry, U.S. Department of Health and Human Services, 1995.

Don Colbert, M.D., was born in Tupelo, Mississippi. He attended Oral Roberts School of Medicine in Tulsa, Oklahoma, where he received a bachelor of science degree in biology in addition to his degree in medicine. Dr. Colbert completed his internship and residency with Florida Hospital in Orlando, Florida. He is board certified in family practice and has received extensive training in nutritional medicine.

If you would like more
information about natural and
divine healing, or information about
Divine Health Nutritional Products,
you may contact
Dr. Colbert at:

Dr. Don Colbert
1908 Boothe Circle
Longwood, FL 32750
Telephone: 407-331-7007
(For ordering product only)
Dr. Colbert's Web site is
www.drcolbert.com.

Disclaimer: Dr. Colbert and the staff of Divine Health Wellness Center are prohibited from addressing a patient's medical condition by phone, facsimile or e-mail. Please refer questions related to your medical condition to your own primary care physician.